Practicals in Microbiology

Practicals in Microbiology

Manideepa SenGupta
MBBS MD (UCM-IPGMER)
Professor and Head
Department of Microbiology
Medical College, Kolkata
Kolkata, West Bengal, India

Mallika Sengupta
MBBS MD (CMC, Vellore)
Consultant Microbiologist
Desun Hospital and Heart Institute
Kolkata, West Bengal, India

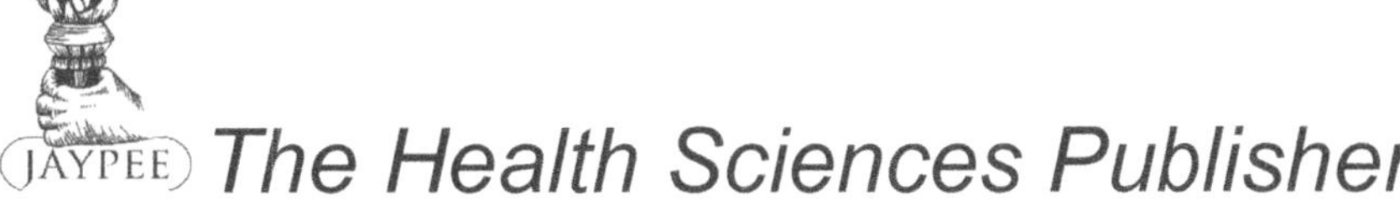

New Delhi | London | Philadelphia | Panama

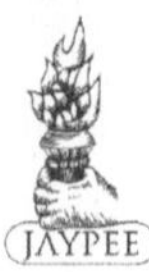

Jaypee Brothers Medical Publishers (P) Ltd

Headquarters

Jaypee Brothers Medical Publishers (P) Ltd
4838/24, Ansari Road, Daryaganj
New Delhi 110 002, India
Phone: +91-11-43574357
Fax: +91-11-43574314
Email: jaypee@jaypeebrothers.com

Overseas Offices

J.P. Medical Ltd
83 Victoria Street, London
SW1H 0HW (UK)
Phone: +44-2031708910
Fax: +44 (0)20 3008 6180
Email: info@jpmedpub.com

Jaypee-Highlights Medical Publishers Inc
City of Knowledge, Bld. 237, Clayton
Panama City, Panama
Phone: +1 507-301-0496
Fax: +1 507-301-0499
Email: cservice@jphmedical.com

Jaypee Medical Inc
325 Chestnut Street
Suite 412, Philadelphia, PA 19106, USA
Phone: +1 267-519-9789
Email: jpmed.us@gmail.com

Jaypee Brothers Medical Publishers (P) Ltd
17/1-B Babar Road, Block-B, Shaymali
Mohammadpur, Dhaka-1207
Bangladesh
Mobile: +08801912003485
Email: jaypeedhaka@gmail.com

Jaypee Brothers Medical Publishers (P) Ltd
Bhotahity, Kathmandu, Nepal
Phone: +977-9741283608
Email: kathmandu@jaypeebrothers.com

Website: www.jaypeebrothers.com
Website: www.jaypeedigital.com

Inquiries for bulk sales may be solicited at: jaypee@jaypeebrothers.com

Practicals in Microbiology

First Edition: **2016,** Reprint: **2025**

ISBN 978-93-5250-133-5

Printed in India

Preface

Up to the early nineties, microbiology was integrated with pathology and a common practical notebook was used. There were dedicated tutors/demonstrators who taught the subject for years together, discussed among themselves and brought an uniformity.

Microbiology is now a separate subject gaining importance everyday. These days, with frequent promotions and frequent transfers, there has been a lack of uniformity among the laboratory notebooks in different colleges.

This book has, therefore, been written in an attempt to bring uniformity and standardization in laboratory and practical notebook among various medical colleges in India.

Manideepa SenGupta
Mallika Sengupta

Preface

Acknowledgments

At the onset, I would like to thank the Lord Almighty, for His blessings that enabled me to complete this book.

Then, I would like to express my sincere gratitude to my teachers, who have taught me and helped me develop my love for microbiology.

Next, I would like to acknowledge my senior colleagues, who have been my constant source of advice and guidance since my postgraduate days.

After that, I would like to thank my friends and colleagues, who form the huge faculty of microbiology in all the Medical Colleges at West Bengal, for their love and support.

I am also grateful to the staff and students of the different medical colleges where I have spent a part of my teaching career.

I acknowledge with fond remembrance all my doctor friends, who are now experts in various fields of medicine.

On behalf of my daughter, Dr Mallika Sengupta, I would like to thank all the teachers, students and staff of Midnapore Medical College, West Bengal and Christian Medical College, Vellore, Tamil Nadu.

I am grateful to Shri Jitendar P Vij (Group Chairman), Mr Ankit Vij (Group President) and Mr Tarun Duneja (Director–Publishing) of M/s Jaypee Brothers Medical Publishers (P) Ltd, New Delhi, India, for publishing this book. I also would like to acknowledge all the staff of Jaypee Brothers (Kolkata), for giving shape to this book.

Last but not least, I would like to express my deepest gratitude towards my family specially my husband, Sri Partha Sarathi Sengupta, son-in-law Dr Anirban Dasgupta and younger daughter Ms Pallabi Sengupta, for their constant encouragement, patience and love.

Contents

Examined

Name ....

College Roll No. ....

University Registration No. ....

University Roll No. ....

Complete | Complete

Examined

Serial No	Page No	Topic	Signature and Remarks

Serial No	Page No	Topic	Signature and Remarks

SECTION 1

GENERAL BACTERIOLOGY

- The microscope
- Sterilization and disinfection
- Culture media
- Culture methods
- Gram staining
- Ziehl Neelsen staining
- Albert's staining
- Morphology of bacteria
- Tests for bacterial motility
- Antibiotic susceptibility testing

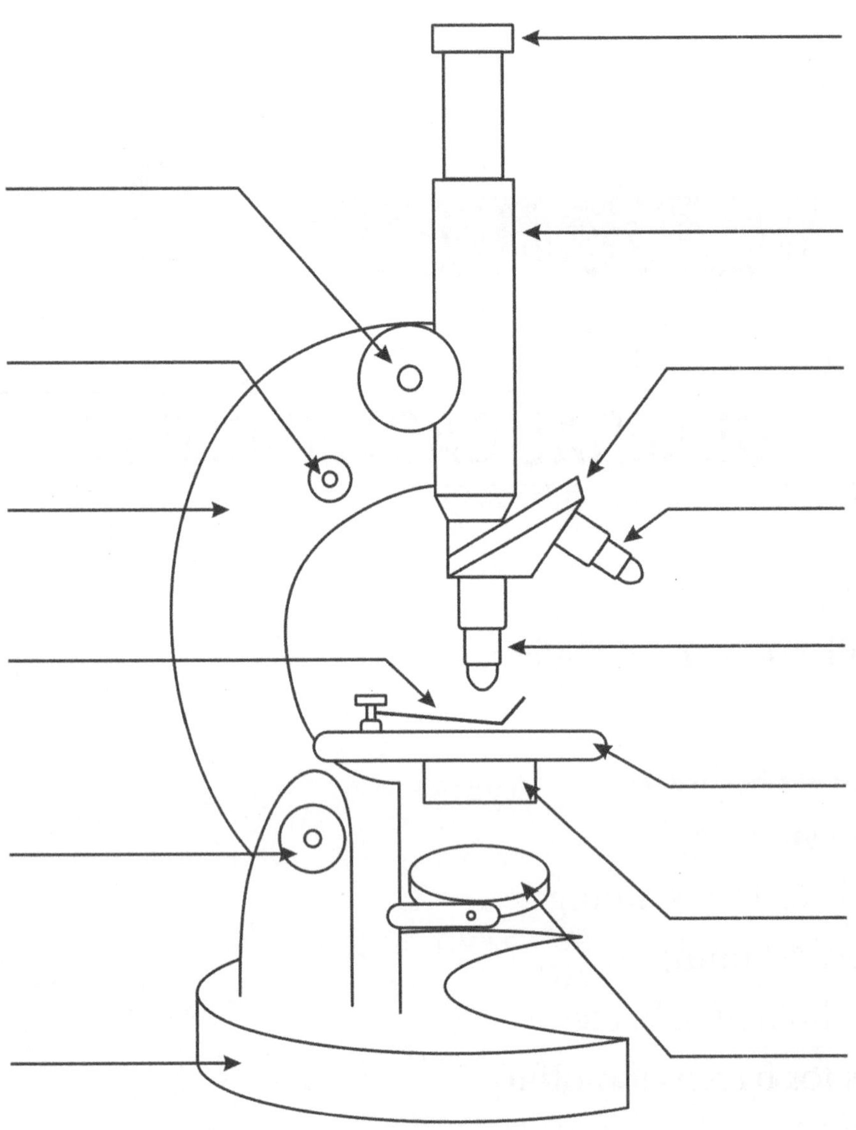

Microscope

1 The Microscope

Definition

The instrument which is used to see an object not visible to the naked eye, by magnifying it, is called a microscope. The most commonly used microscope is a compound microscope.

Parts of a compound microscope

- *Eyepiece*—It enlarges the image produced by the objective but does not improve its quality.
- *Mechanical tube*—It contains the eyepiece at its upper end and nosepiece at its lower end.
- *Focusing adjustment*—Coarse and fine adjustment screw.
- *Nosepiece*—It is attached to the lower end of the mechanical tube. It can be rotated. Three objectives are attached to it.
- *Mechanical stage*—The slide is placed and fixed with clips. It has a central aperture for passage of light. It has two screws for moving the slides.
- *Substage*—It consists of iris diaphragm, condenser and mirror.
- *Iris diaphragm*—It adjusts the amount of light entering into the slide.
- *Condenser*—It regulates the intensity of light falling on the slide.
- *Mirror*—It is plane on one side and concave on the other. It is required for illumination of the object by light reflection.
- *Objective*—These are achromatic lenses which form sharp images. Usually there are three objectives.

Features	*Low power*	*High power*	*Oil immersion*
Focal length	16 mm	4 mm	2mm
Magnification	10X	40X	100X
Mirror used	Concave mirror	Concave mirror	Plane mirror
Iris diaphragm	Closed	Partially open	Fully open
Condenser	Lowered	Lowered	Highest
Use	Initial focusing	Motility Protozoa and helminthic ova	Stained preparation

- *Stand*—It consists of the base placed on the table and arm which is C-shaped holding the mechanical tube and its attachment.

Types of microscope

1. Light microscope—Simple microscope
   Compound microscope.
2. Dark ground microscope—The object appears self-illuminous against a dark background. It has a special dark ground condenser and a central stop.
   Use—Motility of spirochaete is seen.
3. Phase contrast microscope—It is based on the diffraction of light rays. Objects appear dark gray in bright background.
   Use—Study of structure of organism and motility.
4. Fluorescence microscope—It shows fluorescent materials in cells under ultraviolet radiation. Bacteria stained with fluorescent dye appear bright in dark background.
   Use—Auramine O is used to stain *Mycobacterium tuberculosis.*
5. Electron microscope—Object is scanned with high speed electron beam instead of visible light.
   Use—To see virus.
   Types—Transmission electron microscope.
   Scanning electron microscope.
   Confocal laser scanning microscope.
   Scanning probe microscope.

Magnification

It is defined as the increase in length, breadth, diameter of the image in comparison to the object.

Magnification = size of image/size of object
= distance of image from objective/distance of object from objective
= mechanical tube length/focal length of objective

In low power = 160 mm/16 mm (mechanical tube length is 160 mm)
= 10

Hence, magnification in low power is 10 times.

Similarly magnification of high power is 40 and oil immersion is 80 (100) times.

Limit of resolution

It is the minimum distance between two adjacent objects at which they are seen as separate and distinct.

2 Sterilization and Disinfection

STERILIZATION

The process of freeing an article surface or media from all living organisms including bacteria and their spores is called sterilization.

DISINFECTION

It is the destruction or removal of all pathogenic microbes capable of giving rise to infection but not all microbial forms or spores.

ANTISEPSIS

It is the removal of all pathogens from a living surface, e.g. skin.
Sterilization is done by physical and chemical methods.

Physical agents

1. Sunlight
2. Drying
3. Dry heat
   - Flaming
   - Red heat
   - Incineration
   - Hot air oven
4. Moist heat
   - Temperature <100°C
     - Pasteurization
     - Inspissation
     - Vaccine bath
   - Temperature at 100°C
     - Steaming/Tyndallization
     - Boiling

- Temperature >100°C
  - Autoclave

5. Filtration
6. Radiation
7. Ultrasonic and sonic vibrations.

Chemical agents

1. Alcohol
   - Ethyl alcohol
   - Isopropyl alcohol
   - Trichlorobutanol
2. Aldehyde
   - Formaldehyde
   - Glutaraldehyde
3. Dyes
4. Halogens
5. Phenols
6. Surface active agents
7. Metallic salts
8. Gases
   - Ethylene oxide
   - Beta propiolactone
   - Formaldehyde.

STERILIZATION BY DRY HEAT

Mechanism

1. Protein denaturation
2. Oxidative damage
3. Toxic effects of elevated levels of electrolytes.

Heat to red heat

To hold an article in the flame till it is red hot, e.g. inoculating loop/wire, tips of forceps and searing spatulas.

Flaming

To pass an object rapidly through the flame several times without allowing it to become red hot, e.g. glass slide, mouth of test tube, scalpel and needle.

Incineration

For destroying contaminated cloth, animal carcasses and pathological materials.

Hot air oven

- Holding period—160°C for 1 hour.

Precautions

i. Overloading should be avoided
ii. Proper arrangement—To allow free flow of air circulation
iii. Glasswares should be completely dry
iv. Flasks and test tubes should be wrapped in paper
v. It should be allowed to cool down (2 hours).

Uses

- Glasswares, forceps, scissors, scalpels, glass syringes, swabs, liquid paraffin oil, dusting powder, fat and grease.

Disadvantages

i. Hot air—Bad conductor of heat, penetrating power is low.
ii. Fan—Needed for even distribution of air.
iii. Rubber materials and media cannot be sterilized.
iv. If door of oven is opened before room temperature is reached, glassware may crack by sudden or uneven cooling.

Sterilization control

i. Physical—Thermocouples
ii. Chemical—Browne's tube, Bowie Dick tape
iii. Biological—Spores of *Bacillus subtilis*, nontoxigenic *Clostridium tetani.*

STERILIZATION BY MOIST HEAT

Mechanism

1. Denaturation
2. Coagulation of protein.

Pasteurization

- Holder's method—63°C for 30 minutes followed by cooling rapidly to 13°C.
- Flash method—72°C for 15–20 seconds followed by cooling rapidly to 13°C.
- Ultra High Temperature (UHT) Pasteurization—140°C for 3 seconds followed by cooling very quickly in a vacuum chamber.

Use

- Pasteurization of milk.

Inspissation

- Heating at 80–85°C for 30 minutes–1 hour on 3 successive days.

Use

- Sterilization of media containing egg or serum, e.g. Lowenstein Jensen media and Loeffler's serum slope.

Water bath

- Heating at 56°C for 1 hour.

Use

- Serum/body fluids.

Boiling

- Heating at 100°C for 10–30 minutes
- Mostly regarded as means of disinfection.

Precautions

- Materials should be completely immersed, the lid of the sterilizer should not be opened
- 2% sodium bicarbonate may be added to promote sterilization.

Tyndallization

- Arnold or Koch's steamer
- Heating at 100°C for 30 minutes on three consecutive days.

Principle

- Steam at atmospheric pressure—One exposure kills vegetative organisms. Between heatings the spores being kept in a favorable nutrient medium germinate to form vegetative forms which get killed during subsequent heating.

Steaming

- Single exposure at 100°C for 90 minutes may be done.

Use

- Gelatin media and media containing sugars.

Autoclave

Principle

Steam under pressure—Water boils when its vapor pressure is equal to surrounding atmospheric pressure.

When pressure inside a closed vessel increases, the temperature at which water boils is also increased. Saturated steam has high penetrating power. When the steam comes in contact with cooler surface it condenses to water and gives up its latent heat to that surface (1600 ml of steam condenses into 1 ml of water at 100°C and releases 518 calories of heat).

Holding period

121°C for 15–20 minutes at 15 lb/inch^2 pressure.

Uses

Dressings, instruments, lab wares, media and pharmaceutical products.

Sterilization control

- Physical—Thermocouples
- Chemical—Bowie Dick tape
- Biological—Spores of *Bacillus stearothermophilus*.

Radiation

Nonionizing	*Ionizing*
Generates heat	No heat generated—Cold sterilization
Infrared radiation–Mass sterilization of syringes	Gamma and X-rays—Sterilizing plastic syringes, swabs and catheters
UV rays-damages DNA Disinfection of closed areas—Laboratories, operation theaters, biosafety cabinet	*Advantages*: • Effective against viruses, bacteria and bacterial spores • Good penetration of closed packs; items can be prepackaged before sterilization • Heat labile materials can be safely sterilized as no heat is involved
	Disadvantages: • Expensive process • Glass tends to go brown and may be damaged • Damages some types of rubber, PVC, nylon, paper, wood, cotton and metals if irradiated more than once

Filtration

Use

- To remove bacteria from heat labile fluids like serum, sugar solution, urea solution, antibiotics for culture media.

Types

i. Candle filters—It is used for purification of water for industrial/drinking purposes
   a. Chamberland filters made of unglazed porcelain
   b. Berkefeld filters made of fossil diatomaceous earth.

ii. Asbestos filters—These are disposable and single use disks
   a. Seitz filters.

iii. Membrane filters—Cellulose esters
   - Water purification and analysis
   - Sterilization and sterility testing
   - 0.22 mm.

iv. Sintered glass filters
   Made of finely ground glass fused together.

v. High efficiency particle arresters (HEPA).

CHEMICAL AGENTS

Alcohols

- Ethyl alcohol, isopropyl alcohol and methyl alcohol
- Frequently used as skin antiseptics.

Uses

- Hand rubs and hand wash, disinfection of thermometers.

Advantage

- Fast acting and do not leave any residue.

Disadvantages

- Damage lenses, rubber and plastics
- Inflammable.

Aldehydes

Formaldehyde	*Glutaraldehyde (2%)*
Bactericidal, sporicidal, virucidal	Effective against tubercle bacilli, fungi and viruses
Used to preserve anatomical specimens, sterilize metal instruments	Used to sterilize cystoscopes and bronchoscopes, rubber anesthetic tubes, face masks, plastic endotracheal tubes, polythene tubing
More toxic and irritant to the eyes and skin	Less toxic and irritant to the eyes and skin

Dyes

Aniline dye	*Acridine dye*
Brilliant green, malachite green and crystal violet	Proflavine, acriflavine, euflavine and aminacrine
Bacteriostatic	Bactericidal
Inhibited by organic matters	Not affected by organic matters
Used as selective agents in culture media	Less selective

Halogens

Iodine	*Chlorine*
Inhibits protein synthesis and oxidizes –SH groups of amino acids	Hypochlorous acid is an oxidizing agent
Betadine, povidone iodine and Lugol's iodine	Calcium hypochlorite, 10% bleach and sodium hypochlorite
Used as antiseptic	Used as disinfectant

Phenol

Mechanism

- It damages cell membranes, inactivates enzymes and denatures proteins.

Advantages

- Stable, persistent and effective disinfecting agent for materials with organic matter.

Disadvantages

- Leaves residual films, can irritate skin, does not kill endospores, corrosive to rubber and plastics.

Phenols are components of

- Carbolic acid, lysol, chlorhexidine (good skin antiseptic, mouthwash), cloroxylenol (Dettol).

Oxidizing agents

Hydrogen peroxide	*Benzoyl peroxide*	*Peracetic acid*
Act as an oxidant by producing hydroxyl free radicals which attack essential cell components (lipids, proteins and DNA)	Two benzoyl groups linked by peroxide bridge	Hydrogen peroxide + acetic acid
Bactericidal and rapid action	Antiseptic and bleaching agent	Not deactivated by catalase and peroxidases
Disinfection of superficial wounds, contact lenses	Disinfection of skin and treatment of acne	Disinfection of endoscopes

Ethylene oxide

- Colorless liquid, boiling point –10.7°C
- Penetrating gas, sweet ethereal smell
- Highly inflammable (>3% is explosive)
- Action is due to alkylation of protein molecules and reacts with nucleic acid
- Mutagenicity and carcinogenicity
- Effective against various microbes including viruses and spores-sterilizer.

Uses

i. Readily penetrates plastics.
ii. Sterilizes—Heart-lung machines, respirators, sutures, dental equipments, books and clothings, glasswares, metal and paper surfaces and food.
iii. Not suited for fumigating rooms due to its explosive nature.

Surface acting agents

- Widely used as wetting agents, detergents and emulsifiers
- Anionic compounds—Common soap, effective against Gram negative bacteria
- Cationic compounds—Killing effects—It acts on phosphate group of cell membrane.
  For example cetavlon/cetrimide and benzalkonium chloride.

Metallic salt

- Mercuric chloride, mercurochrome, thiomersal and silver salts.
- Copper salts—Fungicide.

3 Culture Media

Definition

An artificial substrate provided with various nutritional requirements for bacterial growth and metabolism is known as artificial culture media.

Classification of media

Consistency

i. Solid
ii. Liquid
iii. Semisolid.

Routine laboratory media

i. Basal or simple media
ii. Enriched media
iii. Selective media
iv. Differential media
v. Indicator media
vi. Enrichment media
vii. Transport media
viii. Anaerobic media.

i. **Basal media**—It is the simplest medium routinely used in laboratory. It contains the basic substances to support the growth of an organism, e.g. nutrient broth, nutrient agar and peptone water.
ii. **Enriched media**—It allows the growth of fastidious organisms because special nutrients like blood, serum, etc. are added to the basal media, e.g. blood agar and chocolate agar.
iii. **Selective media**—It contains substances that inhibit the growth of other organisms thereby helping the growth of the desired organism, e.g. TCBS (thiosulfate citrate bile salt sucrose agar) media for *Vibrio cholerae*.
iv. **Differential media**—It contains certain substances that help in the differentiation of different bacteria based on a property, e.g. blood agar differentiates the different types of hemolysis.

v. **Indicator media**—It contains some substance that changes visibly as a result of metabolic activities of a particular organism, e.g. MacConkey's agar contains neutral red as indicator where lactose fermenters form pink colonies and nonfermenters form pale colonies.
vi. **Enrichment media**—It is always a liquid media that favors the growth of one organism or inhibits the growth of other organisms, e.g. Selenite F broth for *Salmonella sp.*, alkaline peptone water for *Vibrio cholerae.*
vii. **Transport media**—It is used for transportation of specimen like feces, etc. so that the pathogenic organism survives and is not overgrown by the nonpathogenic organisms, e.g. Stuart's media for *Neisseria gonorrhoeae*, Carry Blair media for *Vibrio cholerae.*
viii. **Anaerobic media**—It is devoid of oxygen, has a low redox potential that favors the growth of anaerobes, e.g. Robertson's cooked meat medium and thioglycollate broth.

AGAR AGAR (AGAR FIBER/POWDER)

- It contains long chain polysaccharide, varying amounts of inorganic salts and minute amounts of protein
- It is derived from seaweed
- It is commonly used as solidifying agent.

Agar is used as a solidifying agent because

i. It is nutritionally inert.
ii. It has no color or odor.
iii. It melts at 95°C and solidifies at 42°C, so heat sensitive materials like blood can be added to it at a temperature as low as 45–50°C.
iv. It does not promote or inhibit the growth of any bacteria.
v. Once solidified agar remains unmelted at all temperatures of incubation.

- For solid media—1.5–2% agar is used.
- For semisolid media—0.3–0.5% agar is used.

PEPTONE WATER

Types of media—Basal, liquid.

Composition

i. Peptone—1 gm
ii. Sodium chloride—0.5 gm
iii. Distilled water—100 ml.

Sterilization

Autoclave at 121°C, 15 lb/inch^2 pressure, for 15–20 minutes.

Uses

i. It is used as basal media for preparation of other media
ii. It is used for culture of nonfastidious organism for checking motility
iii. It is used for testing of indole production.

NUTRIENT BROTH

Types of media—Basal, liquid.

Composition

i. Peptone—1 gm
ii. Sodium chloride—0.5 gm
iii. Beef extract—1 gm
iv. Distilled water—100 ml.

Sterilization

Autoclave at 121°C, 15 lb/inch^2 pressure, for 15–20 minutes.

Uses

i. It is used as basal media for preparation of other media
ii. It is used for culture of nonfastidious organism
iii. Used for inoculation for doing antibiotic susceptibility testing
iv. It is used for revival of dormant bacteria
v. It is used for bulk culture of bacteria.

NUTRIENT AGAR

Types of media—Basal, solid.

Composition

i. Peptone—1 gm
ii. Sodium chloride—0.5 gm
iii. Beef extract—1 gm
iv. Distilled water—100 ml
v. Agar—1.5 gm.

Sterilization

Autoclave at121°C, 15 lb/inch^2 pressure, for 15–20 minutes.

Uses

i. It is used as basal media for preparation of other media
ii. It is used for culture of nonfastidious organism
iii. It is used for demonstration of pigment production
iv. It is used for antibiotic susceptibility testing.

BLOOD AGAR

Types of media—Enriched, differential.

Composition

i. Peptone—1 gm
ii. Sodium chloride—0.5 gm
iii. Beef extract - 1 gm
iv. Distilled water—100 ml
v. Agar—1.5 gm
vi. Defibrinated sheep blood—10 ml (conc. varies from 5%–50%).

Sterilization

Nutrient agar is sterilized by autoclaving at121°C, 15 lb/inch^2 pressure for 15–20 minutes. Blood is collected from sheep with sterile precautions.

The sterile nutrient agar is cooled to 45–50°C, defibrinated sheep blood is added to it, mixed well and poured in Petri dish.

Uses

i. It is used for culture of fastidious organisms
ii. It demonstates the hemolytic properties.
  - Alpha hemolysis—*Streptococcus pneumoniae*
  - Beta hemolysis—*Staphylococcus aureus*
  - Gamma hemolysis—*Enterococcus sp.*

CHOCOLATE AGAR

Types of media—Enriched.

Composition

i. Nutrient agar—100 ml
ii. Defibrinated sheep blood—10 ml.

Sterilization

Nutrient agar is sterilized by autoclaving at 121°C, 15 lb/inch^2 pressure for 15–20 minutes and blood is collected from sheep with sterile precautions.

The sterile nutrient agar is cooled to 75°C, defibrinated sheep blood is added to it, mixed well, heated at 75°C in a water bath till it becomes brown in color and then poured in Petri dish.

Uses

It is used for culture of fastidious organism like *Hemophilus sp.* and *Neisseria sp.*

MACCONKEY AGAR

Types of media—Selective, indicator.

Composition

i. Peptone—2 gm
ii. Sodium taurocholate—0.5 gm
iii. Lactose—1 gm (10% aqueous solution 10 ml)
iv. Distilled water—100 ml
v. Agar—1.5 gm
vi. Neutral red 2% in 50% ethanol—0.35 ml.

Sterilization

Autoclave at 115°C, 10 lb/inch^2 pressure for 10 minutes.

Uses

i. It is a selective media for Gram negative bacilli as bile salts are inhibitory to Gram positive organisms.
ii. It differentiates between lactose fermenting and nonlactose fermenting organisms as lactose fermenting organisms produce pink colonies and nonlactose fermenting organisms produce pale colonies.
    - Lactose fermenter—*Escherichia coli, Klebsiella sp.*
    - Nonlactose fermenter—*Salmonella typhi, Vibrio cholerae.*

SUGAR FERMENTATION MEDIA

Types of media—Liquid, indicator.

Appearance—Test tube containing sugar solution with an inverted Durham's tube.

Composition

i. Peptone—1 gm
ii. Sodium chloride—0.5 gm
iii. Distilled water—100 ml
iv. Sugar—1 gm
v. Indicator - Andrade's indicator—1 ml.

Sterilization

Autoclave at115°C, 10 lb/inch^2 pressure for 10 minutes.

Use

It is used for determining fermentation of any sugar with production of acid or acid and gas.

THIOSULFATE CITRATE BILE SALT SUCROSE AGAR (TCBS)

Types of media—Highly selective, differential.

Composition

i. Peptone—1 gm
ii. Yeast extract—0.5 gm
iii. Sodium citrate—1 gm
iv. Sodium thiosulfate—1 gm
v. Ox bile desiccated—0.8 gm
vi. Sucrose—2 gm
vii. Sodium chloride—1 gm
viii. Ferric citrate—0.1 gm
ix. Distilled water—100 ml
x. Agar—1.5 gm
xi. Thymol blue and bromothymol blue 2% in 50% ethanol—0.2 ml each.

Sterilization

Autoclave 115°C, 10 lb/inch^2 pressure for 15–20 minutes.

Use

It is a highly selective media for *Vibrio sp. Vibrio cholerae* ferments sucrose and produces yellow colonies whereas *Vibrio parahaemolyticus* does not ferment sucrose and form green colonies.

LOEFFLER'S SERUM SLOPE

Types of media—Enriched.

Composition

i. Nutrient broth—100 ml
ii. Glucose—1 gm
iii. Sheep or horse serum—300 ml.

Sterilization

Glucose broth is sterilized in autoclave at 115°C, 10 lb/inch^2 pressure for 15–20 minutes. Serum is filtered by Seitz filter and added to glucose broth poured into test tubes and sterilized by inspissation at 85°C for 30 minutes for three consecutive days.

Use

Culture of *Corynebacterium diphtheriae.*

LOWENSTEIN JENSEN MEDIA

Types of media—Selective, differential.

Appearance—Slopes of green-colored media in MacCartney bottles.

Composition

A. Mineral salt solution
   i. Anhydrous potassium dihydrogen phosphate—2.4 gm
   ii. Magnesium sulfate—0.24 gm
   iii. Magnesium citrate—0.6 gm
   iv. Asparagine—3.6 gm
   v. Glycerol—12 ml
   vi. Distilled water - 600 ml.
B. Malachite green solution—20 ml (2% malachite green in sterile distilled water)
C. Egg solution—Fresh unfertilized eggs less than 4 days old—1000 ml.

Sterilization

Mineral salt solution is sterilized in autoclave at 121°C, 15 lb/inch^2 pressure for 15–20 minutes. Eggs are washed with soap and water, dried, cracked with a sterile knife in a sterile beaker and beaten with a sterile egg whisk. It is added to mineral salt solution and malachite green solution and sterilized by inspissation at 80–85°C for 30 minutes for three consecutive days.

Uses

Culture of *Mycobacterium tuberculosis.*

- *Mycobacterium tuberculosis* produces rough, tough, buff-colored dry, irregular and nonemulsifiable colonies.
- *Mycobacterium bovis* produces smooth, white, emulsifiable colonies.

ROBERTSON'S COOKED MEAT BROTH

Types of media—Anaerobic, differential.

Appearance—Meat particles at bottom for 1.5 cm and 4.5 cm of beef infusion broth above it in a glass test tube with cotton plug.

Composition

Cooked meat containing (fresh bullock's heart 500 gm water 500 ml sodium hydroxide 1N 1.5 ml).

The heart is minced and placed in alkaline boiling water, simmered for 20 minutes, filtered, and meat particles dried on a cloth or filter paper.

Peptone infusion broth containing (liquid filtered from cooked meat 500 ml, peptone 2.5 gm sodium chloride 1.25 gm) is prepared.

It is steamed for 20 minutes, HCl is added and pH adjusted to 7.8.

Preparation of complete medium

1.5 cm of meat particles placed in test tube and covered with 4.5 cm broth above it.

Sterilization

It is sterilized in autoclave 121°C, 15 lb/inch^2 pressure for 15–20 minutes.

Uses

Culture of anaerobic organism

It shows the saccharolytic and proteolytic properties of the organism.

- Saccharolytic—Meat turns pink
- Proteolytic—Meat turns black.

DORSET'S EGG MEDIA

Types of media—Enriched.

Appearance—Yellowish white media in screw capped MacCartney's bottle.

Composition

i. Sterile nutrient broth—25 ml
ii. Beaten egg (2–3)—75 ml.

Sterilization

Inspissation at 80–85°C for 30 minutes for three consecutive days.

Use

Subculture and maintenance of *Mycobacterium tuberculosis*.

STERILE COTTON SWAB

Two sterile cotton swabs are placed in glass test tubes.

Sterilization

Hot air oven.

Use

They are used for collection of pus or throat swab from the patient. One swab used for culture and sensitivity while the other is used for smear preparation.

STERILE PLASTIC CONTAINER

Sterilization

Sterilized by ultraviolet/gamma radiation before packing.

Use

It is used for collection of sputum, urine and feces samples.

BLOOD CULTURE BOTTLE

Type of media—Enrichment.

Appearance—Straw-colored liquid in flat medical blood culture bottle.

Composition

i. Nutrient broth
ii. Glucose—0.5%.

Sterilization

It is sterilized in autoclave 115°C, 10 lb/inch^2 pressure for 10–15 minutes.

Uses

Blood culture which is done in—

a. Enteric fever
b. Brucellosis
c. Septicemia
d. Bacterial endocarditis.

Note

Blood culture bottle may contain—

a. Nutrient broth
b. Brain heart infusion broth
c. Trypticase soy broth
d. Bile broth.

4 Culture Methods

Aerobic culture methods

Methods	*Uses*
Streak culture	Isolation of organism
Stroke culture	Subculture of pure growth
Lawn culture	Antibiotic susceptibility testing
Stab culture	Biochemical tests and for keeping stock
Pour plate culture	Estimation of viable count

Anaerobic culture methods

1. Anaerobic media

Robertson's cooked meat media: Discussed before

Thioglycollate broth:

i. It contains reducing substances like sodium thioglycollate, L-cysteine and dextrose
ii. It contains 0.07% agar which retards the convection current
iii. It has a length of 10 cm and maintains anaerobiosis at the bottom
iv. The solution is preheated to remove the dissolved oxygen
v. Resazurin placed at the surface is used as an indicator. It turns red on exposure to oxygen.

2. Candle jar

It is a metallic jar containing the plates. A candle is lit and put inside it and the lid of the jar is closed tightly. The candle burns and uses up the oxygen in the jar thus creating an anaerobic environment inside it.

3. Gaspak

It is commercially available as a disposable envelope which generates hydrogen, carbon dioxide on addition of water. It has a catalyst. It also has an indicator like methylene blue which is colorless in anaerobic condition and turns blue on exposure to oxygen. The plates and gaspak are placed in screw capped jar and an anaerobic environment is created in it.

4. McIntosh and Filde's jar

It is a metallic jar with a metallic lid and has an inlet pipe and outlet pipe which is connected to a suction machine to remove the oxygen. It makes the jar anaerobic by replacing the oxygen with 80% nitrogen, 10% carbon dioxide and 10% hydrogen. Aluminium pellets coated with palladium serve as catalyst.

5 Gram Staining

GRAM STAINING OF BACTERIA

It was introduced by Christian Gram in 1884.

Purpose

It is a differential stain used for classifying organisms into two broad groups—Gram positive and Gram negative. It is also used to see the morphology of the organisms.

Principle

Salton's hypothesis—The Gram positive organisms have a thick peptidoglycan layer which traps the dye—Iodine complex. When decolorizer is added lipid of cell wall of the Gram negative organism is dissolved and the dye moves out. So it takes up the color of counter stain whereas the Gram positive organism retains the primary dye color.

Differences between Gram positive and Gram negative cell wall

Features	*Gram positive cell wall*	*Gram negative cell wall*
Peptidoglycan layer	Thick	Thin
Lipopolysaccharide	Absent	Present
Teichoic acid	Present	Absent
Stain	Primary stain	Counter stain

Smear making

i. A clean grease-free glass slide is taken and labelled.
ii. A drop of normal saline is placed on it.
iii. A colony is picked up with a loop and emulsified in the saline to make a thin uniform smear.
iv. It is air dried, heat fixed and the smear is encircled on the opposite side. This helps in identifying the side of the smear and also shows that the smear is heat fixed.

Components of Gram stain

- Primary stain—Crystal violet, methyl violet or gentian violet
- Gram's iodine—Acts as mordant
- Decolorizer—Acetone (100%)/alcohol (95%)/acetone-alcohol mixture
- Counterstain—Safranine.

Procedure

i. The smear is flooded with crystal violet and allowed to stand for 1 minute
ii. The stain is poured off and the smear is washed with water
iii. It is then flooded with Gram's iodine solution and kept for 2 minutes
iv. It is poured off and washed with water
v. The slide is decolorized with acetone or alcohol for 10–30 seconds and washed with water
vi. It is then stained with counterstain safranine for 1 minute
vii. The slide is washed well with water and air dried
viii. It is seen under oil immersion of the microscope.

Observation

- Gram positive organisms appear purple in color
- Gram negative organisms appear pink in color.

Precautions

i. In old culture, organisms may appear Gram variable
ii. The smear should not be over decolorized as then Gram positive organism may appear Gram negative.

Examples

- Gram positive cocci—*Staphylococcus aureus, Streptococcus pyogenes*
- Gram negative cocci—*Neisseria meningitidis, Neisseria gonorrhoeae*
- Gram positive bacilli—*Bacillus anthracis, Corynebacterium diphtheriae*
- Gram negative bacilli—*Escherichia coli, Pseudomonas aeruginosa.*

6 Ziehl Neelsen Staining

It is a modification of Ehrlich's original method of staining for acid-fast organisms.

Principle

The presence of mycolic acid and lipids of higher fatty acids in intact cell wall are required to make a bacteria acid fast. High lipid content makes the cell wall less permeable and hence once the hot carbol fuchsin enters, it cannot be removed with acid or alcohol. So these organisms are called acid-fast organisms.

Procedure

i. 5 ml of dilute carbol fuchsin taken in a test tube is heated gently till steam arises.
ii. The smear is flooded with hot carbol fuchsin and heated with a Bunsen burner intermittently for 8-10 minutes.
iii. The stain is then poured off and the slide is washed with water.
iv. The smear is then decolorized well with 20% sulfuric acid or 3% acid alcohol until a faint pink color is seen in transmitted light (appears colorless by naked eye).
v. It is the washed with water.
vi. Methylene blue solution is poured on the smear and kept for 2 minutes.
vii. It is poured off and washed with water.
viii. The smear is air dried and observed under oil immersion lens.

Observation

- Acid fast organisms appear bright red in color.
- Non acid-fast organisms are blue due to the counterstain.

Precautions

i. The carbol fuchsin should not be boiled or overheated. The slide should not become dry
ii. Decolorization should be adequate
iii. The slide should be cooled before washing after heating the carbol fuchsin to prevent the cracking of slide.

Acid-fast organisms—examples

- *Mycobacterium tuberculosis*—Slender, curved pink beaded organism
- *Mycobacterium leprae*
- Atypical mycobacteria
- Nocardia
- Spores of bacteria
- Oocysts of cryptosporidium and isospora.

Modifications of Ziehl Neelsen staining

Organisms	*Decolorizer*
Mycobacterium tuberculosis	20% sulfuric acid
Mycobacterium leprae	5% sulfuric acid
Nocardia	1% sulfuric acid
Spores of bacteria	0.5% sulfuric acid
Oocysts of cryptosporidium and isospora	1% sulfuric acid
Brucella sp.	Acetic acid

RNTCP grading of tuberculosis smears

Number of AFB	*Result*	*Grading*	*Number of fields examined*
≥ 10AFB/oil field	Positive	3+	20
1-10AFB/ oil field	Positive	2+	50
10-99AFB/100 oil field	Positive	1+	100
1-9AFB/100 oil field	Record exact number	Scanty	100
No AFB	Negative	Negative	100

Other stains for mycobacteria

- Auramine O stain.

7 Albert's Staining

Principle

It is used for staining of metachromatic granules of *Corynebacterium diphtheriae*. Metachromasia is the property by which the granules take up a different color from that of the body of the bacilli when stained with the same stain. The granules are made up of polymerized metaphosphate and serve as storage granules. The metachromatic granules are also known as Babes Ernst bodies, volutin granules and polar bodies.

Components

- Albert I—Malachite green and toluidine blue
- Albert II—Iodine and potassium iodide.

Procedure

i. The smear is flooded with Albert I and kept for 5 minutes
ii. The stain is poured off and the smear is washed with water
iii. It is then flooded with Albert II and kept for 3 minutes
iv. The stain is poured off and washed with water
v. The smear is air dried and seen under oil immersion objective.

Observation

- The body of the bacilli stain green with the metachromatic granules blue-black in color at the ends
- *Corynebacterium diphtheriae*—It has abundant granules and are arranged in cuneiform arrangement
- Diphtheroids—It has no or few granules and arranged in palisade pattern.

Other stains for metachromatic granules

- Ponder's stain—Blue bacilli with pink granules
- Neisser's stain—Pink bacilli with brown granules.

8 Morphology of Bacteria

STAPHYLOCOCCUS AUREUS

- Gram positive spherical cocci
- Arranged in clusters as the cells divide in three perpendicular planes and daughter cells tend to remain together
- No spores.

STREPTOCOCCUS PYOGENES

- Gram positive spherical or slightly oval cocci
- Arranged in chains as the cells divide in one plane
- No spores.

STREPTOCOCCUS PNEUMONIAE

- Gram positive lanceolate-shaped diplococci, capsulated
- Arranged in pairs
- Long axis of the cocci parallel to the line joining the two cocci
- No spores.

ENTEROCOCCUS FAECALIS

- Gram positive oval-shaped cocci
- Arranged in pairs and short chains
- No spores.

NEISSERIA MENINGITIDIS

- Gram negative cocci
- D-shaped with flat ends apposing each other
- Long axis of the cocci perpendicular to the line joining the two cocci
- No spores.

NEISSERIA GONORRHOEAE

- Gram negative cocci
- Kidney shaped with concave sides facing each other
- Long axis of the cocci perpendicular to line joining the cocci
- No spores.

CLOSTRIDIUM TETANI

- Gram positive bacilli
- Round terminal bulging spore
- Drum stick appearance.

BACILLUS SUBTILIS

- Gram positive bacilli
- Round or oval nonbulging central spore
- Arranged in short chains.

CORYNEBACTERIUM DIPHTHERIAE

- Gram positive bacilli
- Arranged in cuneiform or Chinese-letter pattern (X,V forms)
- Albert stain-green bacilli with bluish black granules.

VIBRIO CHOLERAE

- Gram negative bacilli
- Comma-shaped, curved.

TREPONEMA PALLIDUM

- Silver staining as they are slender
- Spiral coiled bacilli brown color in yellow background.

9 Tests for Bacterial Motility

Definition

Motility is the active movement of bacteria, i.e. displacement from one point to another. It should be differentiated from Brownian motion and flow of bacteria in wet mount.

Tests for motility

1. Hanging drop preparation
2. Unstained wet preparation
3. Semisolid agar
4. Swarming
5. U tube method
6. Craigie's tube method
7. Dark ground microscopy
8. Use of antiflagellar antisera.

Hanging drop preparation

Materials required

- i. A clean dry grease-free glass slide
- ii. Coverslip
- iii. Paraffin/plasticin
- iv. Culture of bacteria
- v. Inoculating loop.

Procedure

1. A clean coverslip is taken and a little amount of paraffin or plasticin is put on the four sides of it.
2. One or two drops of the liquid culture of the bacteria are placed on the center of the coverslip with a sterile inoculating loop. Alternatively one or two colonies of solid culture are suspended in two to three drops of normal saline.
3. A clean, dry grease-free glass slide is placed over the coverslip preparation in such a way that it touches the paraffin layer only.
4. The slide is then turned over such that the culture drop is hanging from the coverslip.
5. It is first seen under low power and then high power objective of microscope.

Observation

The bacteria are seen to be motile or nonmotile at the edge of the drop (air water interface).

Precautions

1. The hanging drop should not be dry and is observed immediately
2. Care should be taken not to press the slide while putting it on the coverslip.

Motile bacteria

Pseudomonas aeruginosa, Escherichia coli.

Nonmotile bacteria

Klebsiella sp., Shigella sp.

Types of motility

1. Darting motility—*Vibrio cholerae*
2. Serpentine motility—*Salmonella sp.*
3. Tumbling motility—*Listeria sp.*
4. Falling leaf motility—Giardia
5. Corkscrew motility—Spirochaete.

Semisolid agar

- Media contains 0.3% agar
- A single stab inoculation is done
- Motile bacteria turns the media hazy
- Nonmotile bacteria grow along the stab line.

Swarming

Seen in *Proteus sp.*

Craigie's tube method

It is used for identification of biphasic flagellar antigen in *Salmonella sp.*

U tube method

Bacteria inoculated through one arm of u tube containing semisolid agar can be subcultured from the other arm if they are motile.

10 Antibiotic Susceptibility Testing

Purpose

To determine the susceptibility or resistance of an isolated organism to a drug.

Methods

1. Diffusion method
   a. Disk diffusion—
      i. Kirby-Bauer method
      ii. Stokes method.
   b. Epsilometer (E-test).
2. Dilution method
   a. Agar dilution method
   b. Broth dilution method.

Kirby-Bauer disk diffusion method

Materials required

i. Media—Mueller Hinton agar (MHA)
ii. Filter paper disk 6 mm along with antibiotic solution or commercial disks that are available
iii. Sensitivity loop
iv. Cotton swab
v. Bacterial suspension
vi. MacFarland's standard.

Procedure

i. The inoculum is first prepared by taking 8–10 colonies from a pure culture, inoculating them in nutrient broth and incubating at 37°C for 2 hours.
ii. The turbidity of the suspension is matched with MacFarland's standard and diluted with normal saline if necessary.
iii. A sterile cotton swab is dipped in the inoculum and plated evenly on a MHA plate as a lawn culture.
iv. Commercial disks are put with sterile forceps. Antibiotic solution is touched with the sensitivity loop, added to the sterile paper disk and put on the lawn culture.
v. All the disks are put at equal distance.
vi. The plate is incubated at 37°C for 16–18 hours.

Observation

The zone of inhibition is measured with a scale and interpreted according to the CLSI guidelines as susceptible, intermediate and resistant.

MacFarland's standard

It contains barium sulfate. 0.5 standard is used for Gram negative bacilli and 1 standard is used for Gram positive cocci.

SECTION 2

SYSTEMATIC BACTERIOLOGY

- *Staphylococcus aureus*
- Coagulase test
- Coagulase negative staphylococcus
- *Streptococcus pyogenes*
- *Bacillus subtilis*
- Biochemical reactions
- *Escherichia coli*
- *Klebsiella sp.*
- *Proteus mirabilis*
- *Proteus vulgaris*
- *Salmonella typhi*
- *Salmonella paratyphi A*
- *Shigella sp.*
- *Pseudomonas aeruginosa*
- *Vibrio cholerae*

11 Staphylococcus Aureus

- **Colony morphology on nutrient agar**—1–2 mm circular, entire, smooth, low convex, opaque colonies with golden yellow pigment.
- **Colony morphology on blood agar**—1–2 mm circular, entire, smooth, low convex, opaque, cream-colored, β-hemolytic colonies.
- **Gram staining**—Gram positive spherical cocci in clusters.

Biochemical reactions

- Catalase test—Positive
- Coagulase test—Positive.

Diagnosis

Staphylococcus aureus.

Other biochemical tests

- Mannitol—Fermented
- Deoxyribonuclease test—Positive
- Phosphatase test—Positive.

MRSA (Methicillin resistant *Staphylococcus aureus*)

- Resistant to many antimicrobials particularly β lactams, aminoglycosides, etc.
- Plays important role in hospital infections.
- Mechanism—Alteration of Penicillin Binding Protein (PBP to PBP2a), excess β-lactamase production, mediated by mec A gene.
- Diagnosis—Disk diffusion method with cefoxitin.
- Screening for carriers—Nasal, axillary and perineal swab.
- Treatment—Invasive infections—Vancomycin and tigicycline.
- Treatment—For carriers—Local mupirocin/bacitracin and chlorhexidine wash.
- Prevention—Handwashing.

12 Coagulase Test

SLIDE COAGULASE TEST

Principle

It detects bound coagulase (clumping factor). It binds to fibrinogen present in plasma and organism aggregates to form clumps.

Procedure

i. A clean dry glass slide is taken and divided into two by a glass marking pencil. The two halves are marked as T (test) and C (control).
ii. A suspension of the colony is made in normal saline on both the halves.
iii. Positive and negative control suspensions may be made.
iv. A drop of undiluted rabbit or human plasma is added to the test side. The other side acts as saline control to note that the organism is not autoagglutinable.

Observation

- Positive—Clumping in 10 seconds
- Negative—Uniform suspension.

Precaution

Autoagglutination if present invalidates the test.

TUBE COAGULASE TEST

Principle

It detects free coagulase. Coagulase is enzyme-like protein which clots plasma in presence of coagulase reacting factor (CRF). Coagulase reacts with CRF and binds to prothrombin, and converts fibrinogen to fibrin.

Procedure

i. Test organism, known positive and negative controls are inoculated overnight in nutrient broth.
ii. 1 ml of 1 : 6 diluted plasma is taken and 0.1 ml of the test organism is put in it
iii. It is incubated at 37°C for 2–4 hours
iv. Positive and negative controls are also tested in the same way.

Observation

- First the positive and negative controls are checked and then the test organism reading is taken
- Positive—Jellification
- Negative—Liquid.

13 Coagulase Negative Staphylococcus

- **Colony morphology on nutrient agar**—1–2 mm circular, entire, smooth, low convex, opaque white colonies.
- **Colony morphology on blood agar**—1–2 mm circular, entire, smooth, low convex, opaque, nonhemolytic white colonies.
- **Gram staining**—Gram positive spherical cocci in clusters.

Biochemical reactions

- Catalase test—Positive
- Coagulase test—Negative.

Diagnosis

Coagulase negative staphylococcus.

Diseases caused

- *Staphylococcus saprophyticus* (novobiocin resistant)—Urinary tract infection
- *Staphylococcus epidermidis* (novobiocin sensitive)—Prosthesis infections.

14 Streptococcus Pyogenes

- **Colony morphology on blood agar**—0.5–1 mm circular, entire, smooth, low convex, opaque, β-hemolytic colonies with wide zone of hemolysis.
- **Colony on nutrient agar**—No growth is seen as it is a fastidious organism.
- **Gram staining**—Gram positive spherical cocci in chains.
- **Catalase test**— Negative.

Diagnosis

Streptococcus pyogenes.

Test	*Group A*	*Group B*
Bacitracin susceptibility	Susceptible	Resistant
CAMP test	–	+
PYRase	+	–
DNAse	+	–
Streptolysin O	+	–
VP test	–	+
Ribose	–	+
Raffinose	–	+
Sorbitol	–	+
Hippurate hydrolysis	–	+

Soluble hemolysin test

Principle

To test for oxygen labile hemolysin streptolysin O.

Procedure

i. The organism is grown in Todd-Hewitt broth overnight.
ii. 0.5 ml of the overnight growth is added to 0.5 ml of 5% washed sheep RBC.
iii. It is incubated at 37°C for 2 hours checking it every 15 minutes to look for hemolysis.
iv. Positive control (which is a known *Streptococcus pyogenes* strain) and negative control (which is *Streptococcus agalactiae*) and RBC control are put up.

Observation

- Positive—Hemolysis
- Negative—Button formation of RBC at the bottom.

15 Bacillus Subtilis

- **Colony morphology on nutrient agar**—1–3 mm, circular, entire, smooth, flat, opaque, dry and grayish colonies.
- **Gram staining**—Gram positive aerobic spore bearing bacilli in short chains.
- **Hanging drop**—Motile bacilli.

Bacillus anthracis	*Bacillus subtilis*
Nonmotile	Motile
Capsulated	Noncapsulated
Penicillin susceptible	Penicillin resistant
Grow in long chains	Grow in short chains
Inverted fir tree in gelatin stab	Rapid liquefaction of gelatin stab
Medusa head colony	Absent
Nonhemolytic	Hemolytic

16 Biochemical Reactions

CATALASE TEST

Principle: It shows the ability of an organism to produce the enzyme catalase. Catalase breaks down hydrogen peroxide to water and nascent oxygen.

Procedure

i. A clean glass slide is taken
ii. A suspension of the colony from an overnight culture with normal saline is made
iii. Positive control and negative control are put up
iv. A drop of 3% hydrogen peroxide is taken and put on the suspension with a Pasteur pipette.

Observation

- Positive—Prompt effervescence or bubbles of nascent oxygen
- Negative—No bubbles.

OXIDASE TEST

Principle: The organism produces the enzyme cytochrome oxidase

Reagent: Tetramethyl para-phenylene diamine dihydrochloride.

Procedure

i. Two to three drops of freshly prepared oxidase reagent is put on a filter paper placed on a Petri dish
ii. One colony of the culture is picked with a glass slide and streaked on the filter paper
iii. Positive and negative controls are tested.

Observation

- Positive—It turns purple immediately within 10 to 30 seconds
- Negative—No color change.

Precautions

i. The oxidase reagent should be freshly prepared
ii. The culture should be fresh and from basal media
iii. Iron rod or loop should not be used to pick up the colony.

INDOLE PRODUCTION TEST

Principle—It demonstrates the ability of a bacteria to produce indole from tryptophan by the enzyme tryptophanase.
Reagent—Kovac's reagent containing para-dimethylaminobenzaldehyde, conc. HCl, amyl or isoamyl alcohol.
Media—Peptone water.

Procedure

Peptone water is inoculated and incubated at 37°C for 24 hours. Kovac's reagent is added to it.

Observation

- Positive—Pink ring on top in the alcohol layer
- Negative—No color development.

METHYL RED TEST

Principle—It demonstrates the ability of a bacteria to produce sufficient acid during fermentation of glucose and maintenance of stable acidity at a pH below 4.5.
Reagent—Methyl red reagent.
Media—Glucose phosphate broth.

Procedure

Media is inoculated and incubated at 37°C for 48 hours. MR reagent is added to it.

Observation

- Positive—Red color
- Negative—Yellow color/no color.

VOGES PROSKAUER TEST

Principle—It demonstrates the ability of a bacteria to produce acetyl methyl carbinol and its reduction product 2, 3-butylene glycol from glucose phosphate in an old culture and maintenance of a stable neutral pH.
Reagent—1 ml of 40% KOH and 3 ml of 5% α-naphthol in absolute alcohol.
Media— Glucose phosphate broth.

Procedure

Media is inoculated and incubated at 37°C for 48 hours. VP reagent is added and shaken well.

Observation

- Positive—Pink color in 2–5 minutes becoming crimson in 30 minutes
- Negative—No color change.

CITRATE UTILIZATION TEST

Principle—It demonstrates the ability of a bacteria to utilize citrate as the sole source of carbon with resulting alkalinity.
Media—Simmon's citrate agar.

Procedure

Media is inoculated and incubated at 37°C for upto 48 hours.

Observation

- Positive—Color turns blue and growth appears
- Negative—No color change and no growth.

Precaution

A light inoculum should be given.

UREASE TEST

Principle—It demonstrates the ability of a bacteria to decompose urea to ammonia and carbon dioxide with the help of enzyme urease.
Media—Christensen's urea medium containing phenol red as indicator.

Procedure

Media is inoculated and incubated at 37°C. Reading is taken immediately, after 4 hours and after 24 hours.

Observation

- Positive—Deep pink color
- Negative—Yellow color.

Precaution

A heavy inoculum should be given.

PHENYLALANINE DEAMINASE TEST

Principle—It demonstrates the ability of a bacteria to deaminate phenylalanine and produce phenyl pyruvic acid.
Reagent—10% ferric chloride.
Media—Phenylalanine agar.

Procedure

Media is inoculated and incubated at 37°C for 4–24 hours. A few drops of ferric chloride is allowed to run down the slope.

Observation

- Positive—A green color in the slope and fluid
- Negative—No green color.

FERMENTATION OF SUGARS

Principle—It demonstrates the ability of a bacteria to ferment a particular sugar with production of acid or acid and gas.
Media—Peptone water with 0.5% sugar and Andrade's indicator. A Durham's tube completely filled with the same liquid is inverted in the media. It is inoculated and incubated at 37°C for 24 hours.

Observation

- Positive—Pink color with or without gas in Durham's tube
- Negative—Colorless.

NITRATE REDUCTION TEST

Principle—It demonstrates the ability of a bacteria to reduce nitrates to nitrites by the enzyme nitrate reductase.
Reagent—Solution A is sulfanilic acid in 5N acetic acid. Solution B is a α-naphthylamine in 5N acetic acid. Just before use solution A and B are mixed in equal volumes.
Media—Potassium nitrate broth.

Procedure

Media is inoculated and incubated at 37°C for 24–48 hours. 0.1 ml of the test reagent is added to it.

Observation

- Positive—Red color within a few minutes
- Negative—No color change.

17 Escherichia Coli

- **Colony morphology on MacConkey agar**—1–2 mm, circular, entire, smooth, low convex, opaque, moist pink lactose fermenting colonies.
- **Gram staining**—Gram negative slender, nonsporing bacilli.
- **Hanging drop**—Motile bacilli.

Biochemical reactions

- Indole production test—Positive
- Urease production test—Negative
- Glucose fermentation—Acid and gas
- Lactose fermentation—Acid and gas
- Mannitol fermentation—Acid and gas.

Diagnosis

Escherichia coli.

Other tests

- Catalase test—Positive
- Oxidase test—Negative
- Methyl red test—Positive
- Voges Proskauer test—Negative
- Citrate utilization test—Negative
- TSI media—Acid slant, acid butt, gas produced and no H_2S.

Diseases caused—Urinary tract infection, diarrhea, meningitis and sepsis.
Diarrheagenic *E. coli*—Salient features:

EPEC	*ETEC*	*EIEC*	*EHEC*	*EAEC*
Infantile diarrhea	Travellers/children diarrhea	Dysentery	Hemorrhagic diarrhea	Chronic diarrhea
Attaching and effacing	Toxin mediated Stable toxin ST Labile toxin LT	Entry endocytosis Invades adjacent cells	Attaching and effacing Vero toxin mediated	Stacked brick appearance in cell cultures
Self-limiting	Toxin like cholera	Sereny test	HUS in children	

18 Klebsiella sp.

- **Colony morphology on MacConkey agar**—2–3 mm circular, entire, smooth, convex, opaque, mucoid pink lactose fermenting colonies.
- **Gram staining**—Gram negative, short, thick nonsporing bacilli.
- **Hanging drop**—Nonmotile bacilli.

Biochemical reactions

- Indole production test—Negative
- Urease production test—Positive
- Glucose fermentation—Acid and gas
- Lactose fermentation—Acid and gas
- Mannitol fermentation—Acid and gas.

Diagnosis

Klebsiella sp.

Other tests

- Catalase test—Positive
- Oxidase test—Negative
- Methyl red test—Negative
- Voges-Proskauer test—Positive
- Citrate utilization test—Positive
- TSI media—Acid slant, acid butt, gas produced and no H_2S.

Diseases caused—Pneumonia, urinary tract infection, meningitis and sepsis.

ESBL

- Extended spectrum beta lactamase producing organism
- Resistant to—All Penicillins, first, second, third generation cephalosporins and monobactams like Aztreonam
- Inhibited by clavulanate and tazobactam
- Diagnosis by disk diffusion method with cefpodoxime, cetazidime and ceftriaxone
- Treatment—Imipenem, meropenem and cephamycins.

19 Proteus Mirabilis

- **Colony morphology on MacConkey agar**—1–2 mm circular, smooth, low convex, opaque, nonlactose fermenting colonies with fishy odor.
- **Gram staining**—Gram negative nonsporing bacilli.
- **Hanging drop**—Motile bacilli.

Biochemical reactions

- Indole production test—Negative
- Urease production test—Positive
- Glucose fermentation—Acid and gas
- Lactose fermentation—Negative
- Mannitol fermentation—Negative.

Diagnosis

Proteus mirabilis.

Other tests

- Catalase test—Positive
- Oxidase test—Negative
- Methyl red test—Positive
- Voges-Proskauer test—Negative
- Citrate utilization test—Variable
- TSI media—Alkaline slant, acid butt, gas produced and H_2S produced
- Phenylalanine deaminase test—Positive.

Diseases caused—Urinary tract infection, wound and burn infection.

20 Proteus Vulgaris

- **Colony morphology on MacConkey agar**—1–2 mm circular, smooth, low convex, opaque, nonlactose fermenting colonies with fishy odor.
- **Gram staining**—Gram negative nonsporing bacilli.
- **Hanging drop**—Motile bacilli.

Biochemical Reactions

- Indole production test—Positive
- Urease production test—Positive
- Glucose fermentation—Acid and gas
- Lactose fermentation—Negative
- Mannitol fermentation—Negative.

Diagnosis

Proteus vulgaris.

Other tests

- Catalase test—Positive
- Oxidase test—Negative
- Methyl red test—Positive
- Voges Proskauer test—Negative
- Citrate utilization test—Variable
- TSI media—Alkaline slant, acid butt, gas produced and H_2S produced
- Phenylalanine deaminase test—Positive.

Diseases caused—Urinary tract infection, wound and burn infection.

21 Salmonella Typhi

- **Colony morphology on MacConkey agar**—1–2 mm circular, entire, smooth, low convex, transluscent, nonlactose fermenting colonies.
- **Gram staining**—Gram negative nonsporing bacilli.
- **Hanging drop**—Motile bacilli.

Biochemical reactions

- Indole production test—Negative
- Urease production test—Negative
- Glucose fermentation—Acid only
- Lactose fermentation—Negative
- Mannitol fermentation—Positive.

Diagnosis

Salmonella typhi.

Other tests

- Catalase test—Positive
- Oxidase test—Negative
- Methyl red test—Positive
- Voges Proskauer test—Negative
- Citrate utilization test—Positive
- TSI media—Alkaline slant, acid butt, no gas produced and trace H_2S produced.

Diseases caused—Enteric fever and septicemia.

22 Salmonella Paratyphi A

- **Colony morphology on MacConkey agar**—1–2 mm circular, entire, smooth, low convex, transluscent, nonlactose fermenting colonies.
- **Gram staining**—Gram negative nonsporing bacilli.
- **Hanging drop**—Motile bacilli.

Biochemical reactions

- Indole production test—Negative
- Urease production test—Negative
- Glucose fermentation—Acid and gas
- Lactose fermentation—Negative
- Mannitol fermentation—Positive.

Diagnosis

Salmonella paratyphi A.

Other tests

- Catalase test—Positive
- Oxidase test—Negative
- Methyl red test—Positive
- Voges Proskauer test—Negative
- Citrate utilization test—Positive
- TSI media—Alkaline slant, acid butt, gas produced and no H_2S produced.

Diseases caused—Enteric fever and septicemia.

23 Shigella sp.

- **Colony morphology on MacConkey agar**—1–2 mm circular, entire, smooth, low convex, transluscent, nonlactose fermenting colonies.
- **Gram staining**—Gram negative nonsporing bacilli.
- **Hanging drop**—Nonmotile bacilli.

Biochemical reactions

- Indole production test—Variable
- Urease production test—Negative
- Glucose fermentation—Acid only
- Lactose fermentation—Negative
- Mannitol fermentation—Variable.

Diagnosis

Shigella sp.

Other tests

- Catalase test—Positive except *Shigella shiga*
- Oxidase test—Negative
- Methyl red test—Positive
- Voges Proskauer test—Negative
- Citrate utilization test—Negative
- TSI media—Alkaline slant, acid butt, no gas produced and no H_2S produced.

Diseases caused—Dysentery and sometimes diarrhea.

24 Pseudomonas Aeruginosa

- **Colony morphology on nutrient agar**—1–2 mm circular smooth, low convex, opaque colonies with diffusible green pigment.
- **Colony morphology on MacConkey agar**—2–3 mm circular, smooth, low convex, opaque, nonlactose fermenting colonies.
- **Gram staining**—Gram negative thin, nonsporing bacilli.
- **Hanging drop**—Motile bacilli.

Biochemical reactions

- Indole production test—Negative
- Urease production test—Negative
- Glucose fermentation—Negative. Oxidatively broken down to form acid only
- Lactose fermentation—Negative
- Mannitol fermentation—Negative.

Diagnosis

Pseudomonas aeruginosa.

Other tests

- Catalase test—Positive
- Oxidase test—Positive
- Methyl red test—Negative
- Voges Proskauer test—Negative
- Citrate utilization test—Positive
- TSI media—Alkaline slant, alkaline butt, no gas, no H_2S produced, metallic sheen.

Diseases caused—Hospital acquired infection

- Ventilator associated pneumonia
- Urinary tract infection
- Surgical site infection
- Bloodstream infection
- Wound and burn infection.

25 Vibrio Cholerae

- **Colony morphology on MacConkey agar**—1–3 mm circular, entire, smooth, low convex, nonlactose fermenting dew drop colonies.
- **Gram staining**—Gram negative nonsporing curved bacilli.
- **Hanging drop**—Motile bacilli—darting motility.

Biochemical reactions

- Indole production test—Positive
- Urease production test—Negative
- Glucose fermentation—Acid only
- Lactose fermentation—Negative
- Mannitol fermentation—Acid.

Diagnosis

Vibrio cholerae.

Other tests

- Catalase test—Positive
- Oxidase test—Positive
- Methyl red test—Variable
- Voges Proskauer test—Variable
- TSI media—Acid slant, acid butt, no gas, no H_2S produced
- Cholera red reaction—Positive
- String test—Positive.

Disease caused—Cholera

Features	*Classical*	*El tor*
VP test	Negative	Positive
Greig's test	Negative	Positive
Polymyxin B sensitivity	Positive	Negative

SECTION 3

IMMUNOLOGY

- Antigen-antibody reactions
- Latex agglutination test for ASO titer
- Latex agglutination test for RA factor
- VDRL test for syphilis
- Widal test for enteric fever
- Enzyme-linked immunosorbant assay (ELISA)

26 Antigen-antibody Reactions

1. Precipitation
   i. Ring precipitation—Ascoli's thermoprecipitin test and Lancefield grouping of streptococcus
   ii. Slide precipitation—VDRL test for syphilis
   iii. Tube precipitation—Kahn test for syphilis
   iv. Immunodiffusion
      a. Single diffusion one dimension—Oudin
      b. Single diffusion two dimension—Radial—Estimation of C_3, C_4
      c. Double diffusion one dimension—Oakley Fulthorpe
      d. Double diffusion two dimension—Ouchterlony, Elek's gel test.
   v. Electroimmunodiffusion
      a. Counter-immunoelectrophoresis
      b. Rocket electrophoresis
      c. Laurell electrophoresis.
2. Agglutination
   i. Slide agglutination—For shigella and vibrio.
   ii. Tube agglutination—Widal test for enteric fever, Weil-Felix test for rickettsia, cold agglutination for mycoplasma, microscopic agglutination test for leptospira, standard agglutination test for brucella.
   iii. Antiglobulin test—Coombs test.
   iv. Passive agglutination—Latex agglutination.
3. Complement fixation test—Wassermann reaction
4. Neutralization test—Estimation of toxins
5. Radioimmunoassay (RIA)
6. Enzyme-linked immunosorbant assay (ELISA)
   i. Antigen detection—Direct/Sandwich ELISA—HbsAg and rotavirus
   ii. Antibody detection
      a. Indirect ELISA—HIV and HCV
      b. IgM capture ELISA—Dengue
      c. Competitive ELISA—HIV.
7. Immunofluorescent assay
   i. Direct—Antigen detection—HSV and rabies
   ii. Indirect—Antibody detection—ANA and FTA for syphilis.

27 Latex Agglutination Test for ASO Titer

Principle

The latex particles are coated with purified antigen of Streptolysin O. When the latex suspension is mixed with serum containing elevated levels of antistreptolysin O antibody on a slide, the particulate antigen combines with antibody and shows agglutination.

Materials required

i. Patient's serum
ii. Positive control
iii. Negative control
iv. Latex particles coated with Streptolysin O antigen
v. Clean glass slide
vi. Stirrer
vii. Pipette.

Procedure

i. The reagents and serum are allowed to come to room temperature.
ii. One glass slide is taken and divided into three equal parts and marked as test (T), positive control (PC) and negative control (NC).
iii. One drop of patient's serum is transferred to the test area with a pipette. Similarly, one drop each of positive and negative control is also transferred to the slide.
iv. The latex reagent is shaken well. One drop of the latex reagent is added to each of test, positive and negative control.
v. All three are mixed well with stirrer.
vi. The slide is rocked and rotated gently and evenly for 2 minutes and observed.

Observation

- Positive control shows agglutination, i.e. clumping and clearing
- Negative control shows no agglutination
- If the test serum shows agglutinatiom then ASO titer is 200 IU/ml or more.

28 Latex Agglutination Test for RA Factor

Principle

The polysterene latex particles are coated with purified human gammaglobulin. When the latex suspension is mixed with serum containing rheumatoid arthritis factor on a slide, the particulate antigen combines with antibody and shows agglutination.

Materials required

i. Patient's serum
ii. Positive control
iii. Negative control
iv. Latex particles coated with human gammaglobulin
v. Clean glass slide
vi. Stirrer
vii. Pipette.

Procedure

i. The reagents and serum are allowed to come to room temperature.
ii. One glass slide is taken and divided into three equal parts and marked as test (T), positive control (PC) and negative control (NC).
iii. One drop of patient's serum is transferred to the test area with a pipette. Similarly, one drop each of positive and negative control is also transferred to the slide.
iv. The latex reagent is shaken well. One drop of the latex reagent is added to each of test, positive and negative control.
v. All three are mixed well with stirrer.
vi. The slide is rocked and rotated gently and evenly for 2 minutes and observed.

Observation

- Positive control shows agglutination, i.e. clumping and clearing
- Negative control shows no agglutination
- Test may or may not show agglutination after 2 minutes and are accordingly noted as positive or negative.

29 VDRL Test for Syphilis

VDRL stands for Venereal Disease Research Laboratory test. It is a nontreponemal test or standard test for syphilis. It is a slide flocculation (precipitation) test.

It is a qualitative/semiquantitative test.

Materials required

i. Patient's serum
ii. Positive control
iii. Negative control
iv. VDRL glass slide (cavity slide)
v. VDRL antigen—Cardiolipin—Antigen
   Lecithin—Visibility
   Cholesterol—Stability
vi. VDRL rotator.

Procedure

i. The VDRL antigen is prepared fresh before the test
ii. The serum is heated at 56°C for 30 minutes
iii. One drop (0.05 ml) of serum is taken in a VDRL slide
iv. To it 1/60 ml of VDRL antigen is added
v. Similarly positive and negative controls are set up
vi. The slide is rotated at 180 rpm for 4 minutes on a VDRL rotator
vii. It is then observed under the low power of microscope.

Observation

- Negative—Uniformly distributed needle-like crystals
- Positive—Large clumps.

  Any positive reaction is tested with doubling dilution with normal saline to determine the titer.

Advantages

- Titer can be determined
- It can be used for both serum and CSF samples.

Disadvantages

- Batch testing is required
- It requires a microscope for taking the result
- Difficult to perform and needs skill
- RPR test is preferred nowadays.

30 Widal Test for Enteric Fever

Principle

It is a semiquantitative tube agglutination test for detection of antibodies against *Salmonella typhi* somatic 'O' antigen, flagellar 'H' antigen and *Salmonella paratyphi* A and B flagellar 'H' antigens by adding a fixed volume of antigen to serial doubling dilutions of patient's serum.

Procedure

i. Four rows of Kahn tubes, each with seven tubes are arranged and labelled as TO, TH, AH and BH respectively.
ii. 0.9 ml of normal saline (0.85%) is added to the first tube of each row and 0.5ml of normal saline is added to all other tubes.
iii. To the first tube 0.1ml of serum is added and mixed well and 0.5 ml is transferred from it to the next tube and so on. From the last tube 0.5 ml is discarded. This is repeated for all the rows.
iv. The last tubes in each row serve as controls and contain no antigen.
v. For each antigen, one control is set up containing normal saline and antigen only.
vi. 0.5 ml of TO antigen is added to each of the first six tubes in the first row. Similarly, 0.5 ml of TH antigen is added to six tubes in second row, AH in third row and BH in fourth row so that the final dilution in each row are 1/20, 1/40, 1/80, 1/160, 1/320 and 1/640.
vii. It is mixed well and incubated at 37°C overnight and the readings are taken the next day.
(Note - 0.4 ml of antigen and antibody are classically used).

Observation

First the control tubes are seen. They should have no agglutination. Then the readings are taken

- Positive—50% clearing of supernatant and clumping deposited at the bottom of the tube
- Negative—No clumping or clearing.

'O' agglutination	Granular (carpeting with rolled out edges)
'H' agglutination	Floccular fluffy deposit

- End point—It is the highest dilution showing 50% clearing and clumping. Titer is the reciprocal of end point
- Titer ≥80 is taken as significant.

Interpretation

i. Antibodies start rising from 7th day and Widal test may be negative in the first week
ii. Antibodies may be present due to previous infection or immunization
iii. The cut off is determined based on the background antibody titer of the population
iv. Persons on antimicrobial therapy may give false-negative result
v. There may be anamnestic reaction—transient rise of antibody titer in unrelated cases.

31 Enzyme-linked Immunosorbant Assay (ELISA)

Principle

It is a qualitative test for detection of antigen or antibody with the help of vice versa. The enzyme is conjugated with a primary or seconday antibody and produce a color reaction with a specific substrate when there is antigen-antibody reaction. The color developed is measured by spectrophotometry.

Enzyme	*Substrate*	*Chromogen*
Alkaline phosphatase	p-nitrophenyl phosphate	
Horseradish peroxidase	Hydrogen peroxide	Tetramethylbenzidine
Horseradish peroxidase	Hydrogen peroxide	ABTS
Horseradish peroxidase	Hydrogen peroxide	Orthophenylenediamine

Types of ELISA

i. Antigen detection—Direct/Sandwich ELISA—HbsAg and rotavirus
ii. Antibody detection
   a. Indirect ELISA—HIV and HCV
   b. IgM capture ELISA—Dengue, JE
   c. Competitive ELISA—HIV.

Procedure of Indirect ELISA

i. All reagents are brought to room temperature. An ELISA plate is taken and marked. The wells coated with antigen are attached to the plate.
ii. The serum to be tested are diluted appropriately and put in each well and incubated. This is to allow the antigen-antibody reaction to occur.
iii. Positive and negative controls are also tested.
iv. It is washed and conjugate is added and incubated again.
v. It is washed and substrate is added and incubated.
vi. The stop solution is added to stop the reaction.
vii. The reading is taken as OD or optical density by spectrophotometer at 450 nm.

Observation

The positive and negative controls are seen first. Then the readings of the samples are taken. Cut off value is calculated.

1. In all ELISA except competitive ELISA
   - Positive—Color development
   - Negative—No color.
2. In competitive ELISA
   - Positive—No color
   - Negative—Color development.

SECTION 4

MYCOLOGY

- Microscopic examination of fungus
- Yeast and yeast-like organisms
- Dermatophytes
- Aspergillus
- Mucor
- Dimorphic fungus

32 Microscopic Examination of Fungus

KOH PREPARATION

Composition

- Potassium hydroxide—10 ml
- Glycerol—10 ml
- Distilled water—80 ml.

Procedure

i. Epidermal scales, skin scrapings, tissue are put on a clean glass slide.
ii. A drop of 10% KOH is put on it.
iii. A coverslip is put on the drop. The slide is then kept for some time in a Petri dish with wet cotton wool or it is gently heated for digestion of the host tissue.
iv. It is seen under low power and high power microscope.

Uses

It is used as 10–40% concentration. It digests protein debris and dissolves cement substances which holds keratinized cells together. It is used to see the morphology of fungus in direct samples, e.g. skin, tissue, nail, hair, etc.

LACTOPHENOL COTTON BLUE STAIN

Composition

Substance	*Volume*	*Function*
Molten phenol	20 ml	Disinfectant
Lactic acid	20 ml	Preserves morphology of fungi
Glycerol	40 ml	Prevents drying
Cotton blue	0.05 gm	Stain
Distilled water	20 ml	

Procedure

i. The culture of fungus is teased and put on a clean glass slide
ii. A drop of LCB stain is put on it
iii. A coverslip is placed
iv. It is seen in low and high power of microscope.

Uses

It is used to see the morphology of fungus in sample and culture for identification.

33 Yeast and Yeast-like Organisms

Features	*Candida albicans*	*Cryptococcus neoformans*
Colony character of culture on SDA slope	2–3 mm nonmucoid, circular, entire, smooth, convex, opaque, regular, cream-colored, buttery consistency, bacteria like colonies with yeasty odor	2–3 mm mucoid, circular, smooth, entire, convex, opaque, regular, cream-colored, bacteria like colonies
Gram stain	Gram positive oval budding yeast cells	Gram positive spherical budding pleomorphic yeast cells
India ink	Oval budding yeast cells without capsule	Spherical budding pleomorphic yeast cells with capsule seen as a clear unstained halo 2–3 times the cell in dark background
Urease test	Negative	Positive
Morphology	Yeast-like	Yeast

34 Dermatophytes

Features	*Microsporum*	*Trichophyton*	*Epidermophyton*
Sites affected	Skin, hair	Skin, hair, nail	Skin, nail
Macroscopy			
Color	White	White	Yellowish green
Texture	Coarse	Granular	Powdery or velvety
Topography	Flat with radiating margin	Flat	Flat with folded in center, thin periphery
Reverse	Yellow to brown	Yellow to brown	Yellow to brown
Hyphae	Hyaline septate branched hyphae	Hyaline septate branched hyphae	Hyaline septate branched hyphae
Macroconidia			
Number	Many	Few to many	Abundant
Shape	Barrel/spindle	Pencil or cigar-shaped	Club-shaped
Size	7–16 μ	20–50 μ	20–40 μ
Arrangement	Singly	Singly	Singly or in clusters
Wall	Thick rough spiny wall	Smooth, thin, wall	Thin smooth wall
Cells	2–8 cells	3–6 cells	2–5 cells
Microconidia			
Shape	Ovoid	Pyriform or globose	Absent
Number	Few	Many	
Arrangement	Sessile along sides of hyphae	Grape like clusters along side of hyphae	

35 Aspergillus

Features	*Aspergillus fumigatus*	*Aspergillus flavus*	*Aspergillus niger*	*Aspergillus tereus*
Macroscopy				
Color	Bluish green	Yellowish green	Brown to black	Light brown
Texture	Powdery	Velvety	Granular	Velvety
Topography	Flat heaped up in center	Flat	Growth fills entire tube	Flat with heaped up center
Reverse	Cream	Cream	Cream	Tan
Hyphae	Septate hyaline	Septate hyaline	Septate hyaline	Septate hyaline
Width	3–8 μ	5–6 μ	6 μ	5 μ
Conidiophore				
Length	150–300 μ	400–850 μ	400–3000 μ	100–250 μ
Wall	Smooth parallel	Rough parallel	Braoad brown tint	Smooth parallel
Vesicle	Flask-shaped	Globose/ subglobose	Spherical	Dome-shaped
Phialides	Uniseriate	Uniseriate/biseriate	Biseriate	Biseriate
Surface of vesicle covered	Upper half	Most of vesicle	Entire	Upper half
Conidia				
Shape	Round	Round	Round	Ellipsoidal
Size	2–5 μ	4 μ	4–5 μ	2 μ
Arrangement	Compact chains	Loose divided chains	Ecchinulate in compact chains	Long straight chains

36 Mucor

Features	*Mucor*
Macroscopy Color Texture Nature Reverse	 White Wooly Growth in entire tube with dark spot Cream
Hyphae Width	Broad aseptate hyaline 10 μ
Sporangiophore	Long straight
Columella	Round to oval
Collarette	Present at the base of columella
Sporangia	Globose
Sporangiospores	Ovoid

37 Dimorphic Fungus

Features	*Histoplasma capsulatum*
Macroscopy	
Color	White to brown
Texture	Woolly fluffy
Reverse	Yellow
Tissue section	2–5 μ oval yeast cells
Hyphae	Thin septate hyaline
Width	1–2 μ
Conidiophore	Long, slender, right angle to hyphae
Macroconidia	
Shape	Spherical
Size	8–14 μ
Wall	Tuberculate with projections
Microconidia	
Shape	Spherical
Size	2–5 μ
Wall	Smooth

SECTION 5

PARASITOLOGY

- Processing of stool
- Trophozoites and cysts in stool
- Helminth ova
- Morphology of adult worms
- Parasites in blood and bone marrow smear
- Good laboratory practice

38 Processing of Stool

Collection of stool

1. Stool is collected in a clean dry wide mouthed container
2. Stool must be freshly collected
3. Urine should not be allowed to mix with stool
4. Stool is collected before starting medications
5. Barium and bismuth salts for enema and radiological investigations are avoided.

Macroscopy

1. Color
2. Odor
3. Consistency
4. Presence of blood or mucus
5. Adult parasites seen.

Microscopic examination

1. Saline preparation
2. Iodine preparation
3. Staining methods
   - Eosin staining for cysts and trophozoite
   - Modified Ziehl Neelsen staining for *Cryptosporidium sp.*, *Cyclospora sp.*, *Isospora sp.*
   - Modified trichome stain for *Microsporidium sp.*
   - Field's stain for *Giardia sp.*
   - Carmine stain for proglottids of *Taenia sp.*
   - Calcofluor stain for *Acanthamoeba sp.*

NORMAL CONSTITUENTS OF STOOL

i. Food substances—Vegetable cell and vegetable fibers
ii. Cells—Epithelial cell, macrophage and few leukocyte
iii. Crystals—Oxalate crystals.

ABNORMAL CONSTITUENTS OF STOOL

i. Cells—RBC and excess pus cells
ii. Crystals—Charcot-Leyden crystals
iii. Protozoa—Trophozoite and cysts
iv. Helminths—Ova.

WET PREPARATION—SALINE AND IODINE PREPARATION

Materials required

i. Two clean glass slides
ii. Wooden applicator sticks
iii. Normal saline (0.85%) solution
iv. Lugol's iodine solution
v. Coverslip.

Procedure

i. On one clean glass slide a drop of normal saline is placed and on the other glass slide a drop of iodine is placed.
ii. After mixing the stool specimen well with a wooden applicator stick a uniform suspension of stool specimen is made first in saline and then iodine. Care should be taken so that the suspension is neither too thin nor too thick.
iii. A coverslip is placed on each of the suspensions taking care not to introduce any air bubble.
iv. The slides are examined under low power and high power of microscope.

Uses

a. Saline preparation
   i. For detection of cyst and trophozoite in stool
   ii. For seeing movement of trophozoite
   iii. For detection of ova of helminth and classifying them as bile stained or non bile stained.

b. Iodine preparation

For identification of the cysts and trophozoite of protozoa as iodine stains the nuclei and glycogen mass. Protozoa are killed hence motility cannot be seen.

CONCENTRATION METHODS OF STOOL

When only a small number of organisms are present in stool then concentration procedures help in detection of ova and cysts as it allow the bulk of stool to be removed while ova and cysts remain. These methods are—

i. Formol ether sedimentation technique
ii. Saturated common salt floatation technique
iii. Zinc sulfate floatation technique.

FORMOL ETHER SEDIMENTATION TECHNIQUE

Procedure

i. In a 10 ml centrifuge tube, 7 ml of 10% formalin is taken
ii. 1 gm of feces is taken with the help of applicator stick and mixed in the formalin
iii. 3 ml of ether is poured into the centrifuge tube
iv. It is mixed well in a vortex for 5 minutes
v. The tube is then centrifuged at 3000 rpm for 1 minute.
vi. After centrifugation four layers are seen from top to bottom
    - Ether at the top
    - Fecal debris next to ether
    - Formalin forms the third layer
    - Deposit containing ova and cyst at the bottom.
vii. The supernatant is discarded and the deposit is used for making wet preparation and stained smears.

SATURATED COMMON SALT FLOATATION TECHNIQUE

Procedure

i. A small square container with erect sides and straight edge is taken (about 1″ × 1″).
ii. A small amount of stool is mixed well with a few drops of saturated salt solution in the container by stirring with a glass rod.
iii. The container is then filled up with saturated salt solution almost upto the brim, stirring being continued though out.
iv. With the help of a pipette saturated salt solution is put in the container drop-by-drop so that a convex meniscus of the liquid is formed.
v. A clean glass slide is carefully placed on top of the container so that its center touches the liquid.
vi. The whole setup is allowed to stand undisturbed for 30 minutes.
vii. The slide is then quickly turned over, covered with a coverslip and examined under the microscope.

39 Trophozoites and Cysts in Stool

ENTAMOEBA HISTOLYTICA AND *ENTAMOEBA COLI* CYST

Features	*Entamoeba histolytica cyst*	*Entamoeba coli cyst*
Size	10–15 μ	15–30 μ
Shape	Spherical	Spherical
Nucleus	1–4	1–8
Karyosome	Small, compact, central	Eccentric
Chromatoid body	Present, blunt ends	Rare, pointed ends
Glycogen mass	In uninucleate stage	In binucleate stage

ENTAMOEBA HISTOLYTICA TROPHOZOITE

- Size—15–30 μ
- Shape—No definite shape
- Nucleus—Single nucleus
- Karyosome—Central
- Motility—Actively motile
- Cytoplasm—Defined into ectoplasm and endoplasm
- RBC—Presence of ingested RBC in cytoplasm.

GIARDIA LAMBLIA TROPHOZOITE AND CYST

Features	*Giardia lamblia trophozoite*	*Giardia lamblia cyst*
Size	15 μ long, 9 μ wide	8–15 μ long, 6–10 μ wide
Shape	Tear-drop, pyriform, tennis-racket shape	Oval
Symmetry	Bilaterally symmetrical	Bilaterally symmetrical
Axostyle	2, running in midline	2, running in midline
Nucleus	2	4
Parabasal body	2	2
Flagella	4 pairs	Remnants of flagella
Wall	Thin	Tough hyaline
Motility	Falling leaf motility	Nonmotile

40 Helminth Ova

FERTILIZED EGG OF *ASCARIS LUMBRICOIDES*

- Shape—Oval or round.
- Size—60–75 μ long and 40–50 μ wide.
- Color—Bile stained and brown.
- Wall—It is surrounded by a thick shell with outer albuminous coat thrown into mammilations. The mammilations are lost in decorticated eggs.
- Ovum—Large unsegmented ovum.
- Other features—Clear crescentic area present at each pole.
- Floatation in saturated solution of common salt—Floats.

UNFERTILIZED EGG OF *ASCARIS LUMBRICOIDES*

- Shape—Elliptical
- Size—80–90 μ long, 45–55 μ wide
- Color—Bile stained and brown
- Wall—It has a thin shell with irregular scanty mammilations
- Ovum—Small and atrophied ovum
- Other features—A mass of disorganized highly refractile granules of various sizes are present
- Floatation in saturated solution of common salt—Sinks.

EGG OF A *TAENIA SP.*

- Shape—Spherical
- Size—31–43 μ in diameter
- Color—Bile stained and brown
- Wall—Thick and radially striated shell called embryophore
- Ovum—An embryo called oncosphere 14–20 μ in diameter
- Other features—Three pairs of hooklets
- Floatation in saturated solution of common salt—Sinks.

EGG OF HOOKWORM

- Shape—Oval or elliptical
- Size—55-65 μ long, 36–40 μ wide
- Color—Not bile stained and colorless
- Wall—Thin translucent hyaline shell membrane
- Ovum—Segmented ovum with four blastomeres
- Other features—It has a clear space between the shell and the ovum
- Floatation in saturated solution of common salt—Floats.

EGG OF *TRICHURIS TRICHIURA*

- Shape—Barrel-shaped
- Size—50–55 μ long, 20–25 μ wide
- Color—Bile stained and brown
- Wall—Thick double layered shell
- Ovum—An unsegmented ovum
- Other features—Presence of a mucous plug projecting at each pole
- Floatation in saturated solution of common salt—Floats.

EGG OF *ENTEROBIUS VERMICULARIS*

- Shape—Planoconvex
- Size—50–60 μ long, 30 μ wide
- Color—Not bile stained and colorless
- Wall—Transparent shell
- Ovum—A coiled tadpole-like larva
- Floatation in saturated solution of common salt—Floats.

EGG OF *HYMENOLEPIS NANA*

- Shape—Spherical or oval.
- Size—35–45 μ diameter.
- Color—Not bile stained and colorless.
- Wall—Thin colorless outer membrane and an inner embryophore enclosing the embryo. The space between the two membranes contains yolk granules and 4–8 polar filaments.
- Ovum—Hexacanth embryo.
- Other features—Three pairs of hooklets.
- Floatation in saturated solution of common salt—Floats.

EGG OF *HYMENOLEPIS DIMINUTA*

- Shape—Spherical or oval.
- Size—50–80 μ diameter.
- Color—Bile stained and brown.
- Wall—Thin colorless outer membrane and an inner embryophore enclosing the embryo. The embryphore has two knob-like thickenings.
- Ovum—Hexacanth embryo.
- Other features—Three pairs of hooklets.
- Floatation in saturated solution of common salt—Floats.

41 Morphology of Adult Worms

TAENIA SP.

Flat tape-like elongated structure with segments longer than broad.

Features	*Taenia saginata*	*Taenia solium*
Length	5–10 meter	2–3 meter
Scolex	Large, size 1–2 mm quadrate, four suckers, no rostellum, no hooks, suckers may be pigmented	Small, size 1 mm globular, four suckers, rostellum and hooks present, suckers not pigmented
Neck	Long, narrow, fragile	Short, thick
Proglottids	1000–2000	Below 1000
Expulsion of segments	Expelled singly and may force open anal sphincter	Expelled passively in chains of 5–6
Uterus	Lateral branches 15–30 on each side, thin and dichotomous	Lateral branches 5–10 on each side, thick and dendritic
Vaginal sphincter	Present	Absent
Ovaries	2, no accessory lobe	2, with accessory lobe
Testes	300–400 follicles	150–200 follicles
Lifespan	10 years	25 years

CYSTICERCUS

Cysticercus cellulosae is the larval form of *Taenia solium* present in skeletal muscle, brain, lung, heart, liver, etc. This happens when man serves as the intermediate host. It occurs when man swallows *Taenia* eggs with water, raw vegetables or due to unclean or unhygienic personal habits or due to reversal of peristaltic movement in intestine. The larvae penetrate the mucosa and are present in other parts of the body. Symptoms occur according to the site of infection. It is diagnosed by CT scan, MRI and biopsy. *Cysticercus bovis* does not occur in man.

HYDATID CYST

- It is the larval form of *Echinococcus granulosus.*
- It is a cystic cavity formed by the developing embryo.
- It is commonly found in liver (70%), lung (20%), spleen (3%), brain (3%) and other organs like bone, pelvic organs, etc.
- It has three layers covering it, from inside outwards they are—
  1. i. Endocyst—Inner germinal layer.
  2. ii. Ectocyst—Outer laminated layer.
  3. iii. Pericyst—Adventitious fibrous layer formed due to reaction of the host.
- Inside it contains the hydatid fluid secreted by the germinal layer.
- From the wall of germinal layer the brood capsules develop which contain the protos colices with hooks and suckers.
- It is diagnosed by USG and CT scan.

ASCARIS LUMBRICOIDES

- Common name—Roundworm
- Shape—Elongated, round, smooth with tapering ends
- Color—Colorless
- Anterior end is thinner than posterior end
- Nonsegmented worm.

Features	*Male*	*Female*
Size	15–25 cm × 3–4 mm	25–40 cm × 4–5 mm
Posterior end	Coiled	Tapering
Genital opening	At posterior end along with anus forms the cloaca	At the junction of anterior and middle 1/3rd
Spicules	Present	Absent
Papillae	Pre- and postanal—Multiple	Postanal—One pair

ENTEROBIUS VERMICULARIS

- Common name—Pinworm, threadworm
- Shape—Cylindrical, round, smooth with pointed ends
- Color—White
- It has three lips around the mouth surrounded by cuticular expansion
- There is no buccal capsule
- The tegument is transversely striated.

Features	*Male*	*Female*
Size	2–4 mm × 0.1–0.2 mm	8–12 mm × 0.3–0.5 mm
Posterior end	Tightly curved, sharply truncated	Straight with a pin-like tail
Copulatory bursa	Present	Absent
Life span	Short as it dies after fertilizing the female	37–100 days

TRICHURIS TRICHIURA

- Common name—Whipworm
- Anterior 3/5th is thin and hair-like and posterior 2/5th is short and thick giving resemblance to a whip
- Nonsegmented and smooth.

Features	*Male*	*Female*
Size	3–4 cm long	4–5 cm long
Posterior end	Coiled ventrally	Straight, shaped-like a comma

ANCYLOSTOMA DUODENALE/NECATOR AMERICANUS

- Common name—Hookworm
- Cylindrical, nonsegmented and smooth.

Features	*Ancylostoma duodenale*	*Necator americanus*
Size		
Male	8–11 × 0.4 mm	7–9 × 0.3 mm
Female	10–13 × 0.6 mm	9–11 × 0.4 mm
Head end	Bent in the same direction as body	Bent in the opposite direction to the body
Buccal capsule	Elongated and pear-shaped	Spherical
	4 ventral teeth hook-like and 2 dorsal rudimentary teeth knob-like	2 ventral and 2 dorsal cutting plates
Copulatory bursa of male	13 rays, dorsal ray single	14 rays, dorsal ray bipartite
Caudal spine in female	Present	Absent
Vulval opening	At the junction of middle 1/3rd and posterior 1/3rd	At the junction of anterior 1/3rd and middle 1/3rd

DRACUNCULUS MEDINENSIS

- Common name—Guineaworm
- Shape—Cylindrical, smooth, rounded and nonsegmented
- Size—Female: 60–100 cm × 0.9–1.7 mm
- Smooth cuticle
- Posterior end is blunt and bent to form a hook
- Male—2.5 cm × 0.4 mm (rarely seen)
- Female is the longest nematode infecting man.

FASCIOLA HEPATICA

- Shape—It is a large leaf-like fluke (Trematode)
- Size—30 mm × 13 mm
- Color—Brown and pale gray
- It has a spiny tegument
- It has two suckers—The oral is smaller and the ventral is larger
- It has a conical projection at the anterior end.

FASCIOLOPSIS BUSKI

- Shape—It is a large fleshy ovoid fluke (Trematode)
- Size—20–75 mm long, 8–20 mm broad
- It has a small oral sucker and a large ventral sucker
- It has a large acetabulum
- The ventral surface is covered with transverse spines but the dorsal surface is smooth.

42 Parasites in Blood and Bone Marrow Smear

LEISHMAN STAINING

It is a Romanowsky stain which contains Leishman powder dissolved in acetone-free alcohol. It stains the acidic and basic constituents of the cell differently.

Procedure

i. The smear is covered with 10 drops of Leishman stain and kept for 1–2 minute
ii. Double volume, i.e. 20 drops of buffered water is added to the stain and mixed well and left for 10 minutes
iii. The smear is washed with water and air dried
iv. It is observed under oil immersion in the microscope.

PLASMODIUM

The cytoplasm of malaria parasite stain blue while the chromatin stains red in color.

Features	*P. falciparum*	*P. vivax*
RBC Size Other features	 Normal Maurer's cleft	 Enlarged Schuffner's dot
Ring form (early Trophozoites):	1 or more small red chromatin dot. Blue cytoplasm not thicker opposite to the chromatin. Accole form seen. Multiple rings present	Usually single large red chromatin dot. Blue cytoplasm thicker opposite to the chromatin – signet ring appearance. Accole form not seen
Late trophozoites	Compact, vacoulated, Not seen in peripheral blood	Ameboid, central vacoule, light blue cytoplasm
Schizont	18–24 merozoites. Not seen in peripheral blood	12–24 merozoites
Pigment	Dark to black clumped mass	Fine granular yellow brown
Gametocytes	Crescent sausage-shaped	Spherical, compact, fills the cell

LEISHMANIA DONOVANI AMASTIGOTES

- Bone marrow smear
- Intracellular and extracellular Leishman Donovan (LD) bodies
- Shape—Round or oval
- Size—2–4 μ along the longitudinal axis
- Usually found in groups, in or near reticuloendothelial cells
- It contains light blue cytoplasm, large pinkish red nucleus and small red kinetoplast
- The nucleus is round and the kinetoplast is elongated giving it a 'dot and dash' appearance
- Differential diagnosis—Toxoplasma gondii and Histoplasma capsulatum.

MICROFILARIA

Features	*Wuchereria bancrofti*	*Brugia malayi*
Length	250–300 μ	175–230 μ
Breadth	6–7 μ	6 μ
Sheath	Present, lightly stained	Present, deeply stained
Cephalic space	Length and breadth equal	Length is twice the breadth
Nuclear chromatin	Discrete nuclei	Blurred
Tail tip	Free of nuclei	Two nuclei present
Body curve	Regular, sweeping curve	Irregular, kinky curve
Stylet at anterior end	Single	Double
Excretory pore	Not prominent	Prominent

43 Good Laboratory Practice

1. Entry of only authorized persons. No children, pregnant women visitors, animals are allowed in the laboratory.
2. Appropriate signs including universal biohazard symbol should be put.
3. Smoking, drinking, eating are not permitted.
4. Long hair should be tied up and heavy/noisy jewellery, contact lens and cosmetics should be avoided.
5. Immunization is mandatory for workers.
6. Instruments should have proper labeling and safe operation is ensured.
7. Mouth pipetting is strictly prohibited.
8. Use of personal protective equipment (PPE) like gloves, mask, apron is a must.
9. Handwashing prevents transmission of infection.
10. Adequate decontamination before washing or disposing waste with proper waste segregation and disposal should be done.

Index